# TYPE 2 DIABETES COOKBOOK FOR BEGINNERS

*Delicious & Easy Recipes + 30-Day Meal Plan for Beginners*

**T. John**

# COPYRIGHT PAGE

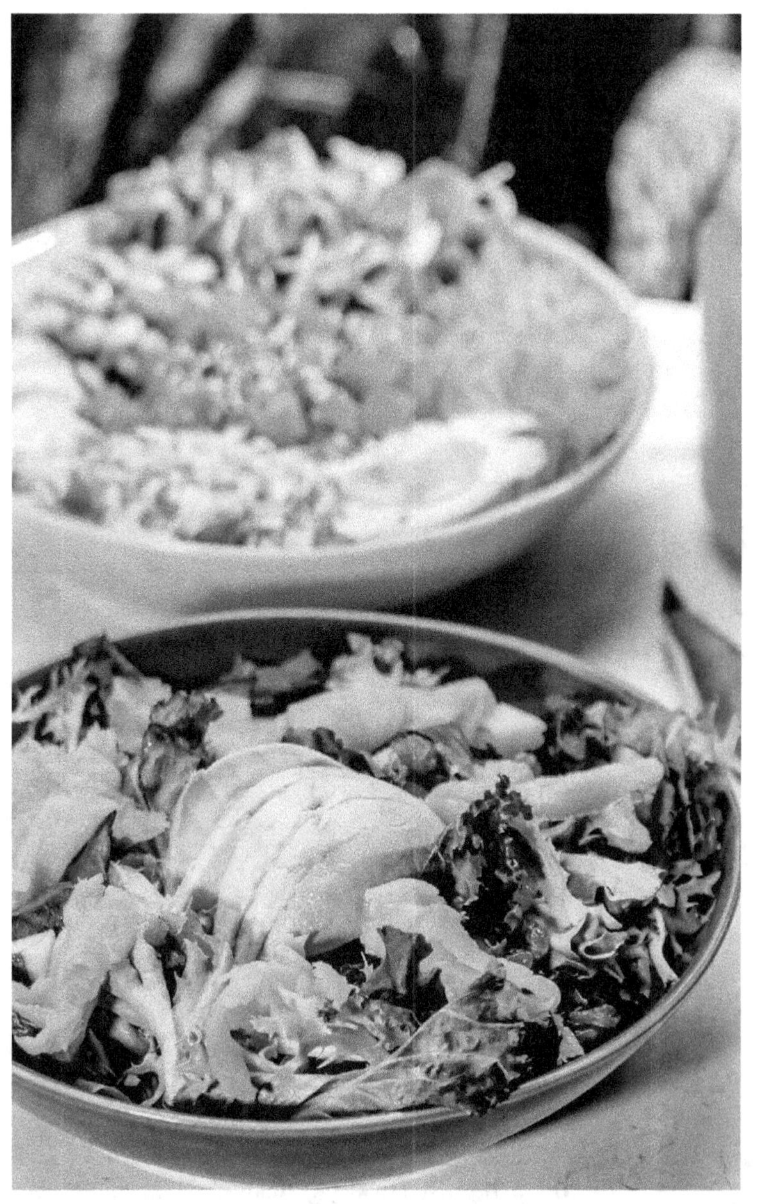

# TABLE OF CONTENTS


**INTRODUCTION** ...................................................9

Understanding Type 2 Diabetes:..................... 9

Importance of a Healthy Diet:...................... 10

Basics of Meal Planning for Diabetes:.......................... 11

**Chapter 2: 30 Day Meal Plan** ........................13

Week 1: ....................................................... 13

Week 2: ....................................................... 15

Week 3: ....................................................... 17

Week 4: ....................................................... 20

**Chapter 2: Breakfast Recipes**...........................24

Quinoa Breakfast Bowl........................................ 24

Vegetable Omelette............................................ 25

Greek Yogurt Parfait.......................................... 26

Chia Seed Pudding............................................. 27

Whole Grain Pancakes ......................................... 28

Avocado Toast with Poached Egg .............................. 29

Berry and Almond Smoothie Bowl............................... 30

Spinach and Feta Breakfast Wrap.............................. 31

Overnight Oats with Berries ................................. 32

Sweet Potato Hash with Turkey Sausage....................... 33

Egg and Veggie Muffins....................................... 34

Cottage Cheese and Fruit Plate ........................... 36

Almond Butter and Banana Toast ....................... 37

Veggie and Cheese Breakfast Quesadilla ..................... 38

Smoked Salmon and Cream Cheese Bagel ................. 39

## Chapter 3: Lunch Recipes ........................................41

Grilled Chicken Salad ................................................ 41

Quinoa and Black Bean Bowl ................................... 42

Turkey and Veggie Wrap ........................................... 44

Lentil Soup ................................................................. 45

Shrimp and Broccoli Stir-Fry .................................... 47

Chickpea and Vegetable Curry ................................. 48

Turkey and Avocado Lettuce Wraps ......................... 49

Caprese Salad with Balsamic Glaze .......................... 51

Grilled Salmon with Asparagus ................................ 52

Zucchini Noodles with Pesto .................................... 53

Chicken and Vegetable Skewers ................................ 55

Spinach and Mushroom Quesadilla .......................... 56

Tomato Basil Soup ..................................................... 57

Cauliflower Fried Rice ............................................... 59

Tuna Salad Lettuce Wraps ........................................ 60

## Chapter 4: Dinner Recipes ...................................... 62

Baked Chicken Breast with Roasted Vegetables .......... 62

Quinoa-Stuffed Bell Peppers .................................... 63

Salmon with Lemon-Dill Sauce ................................ 65

Eggplant and Tomato Gratin.................................. 66

Turkey and Sweet Potato Casserole........................... 67

Stir-Fried Tofu with Broccoli ................................ 69

Spaghetti Squash with Marinara Sauce....................... 70

Teriyaki Chicken Skillet ..................................... 71

Cod with Mediterranean Salsa ................................ 73

Mushroom and Spinach Stuffed Chicken ..................... 74

Beef and Vegetable Stir-Fry .................................. 76

Baked Cod with Lemon and Herbs............................ 77

Butternut Squash and Lentil Curry ............................ 79

Grilled Veggie and Hummus Wrap ............................ 80

Baked Pork Chops with Apple Compote...................... 81

**Chapter 5: Snacks and Appetizers ................84**

Guacamole with Veggie Sticks................................. 84

Greek Yogurt Dip with Cucumber Slices ..................... 85

Mixed Nuts and Seeds ........................................ 86

Cheese and Whole Grain Crackers ............................ 87

Hummus and Carrot Sticks .................................... 88

Cottage Cheese and Pineapple ................................ 89

Edamame with Sea Salt ....................................... 90

Roasted Chickpeas ........................................... 91

Avocado and Tomato Salsa ................................... 92

Apple Slices with Almond Butter .............................. 93

Veggie Spring Rolls........................................... 94

Kale Chips...................................................... 95

Mozzarella and Tomato Skewers.............................. 96

Trail Mix with Dried Fruits.................................... 97

Sweet Potato Fries with Yogurt Dip .......................... 98

## Chapter 6: Desserts ...................................... 100

Berry and Yogurt Parfait..................................... 100

Dark Chocolate-Dipped Strawberries ...................... 101

Baked Apples with Cinnamon ............................... 102

Sugar-Free Pumpkin Pie ..................................... 103

Greek Yogurt Popsicles ...................................... 104

Almond Flour Chocolate Chip Cookies..................... 105

Chia Seed Chocolate Pudding................................ 106

Fresh Fruit Salad ............................................. 107

Avocado Chocolate Mousse ................................. 108

Banana Walnut Muffins ...................................... 109

Ricotta and Berry Tartlets.................................... 110

Mango Sorbet................................................. 111

Pistachio Date Balls .......................................... 112

Peach Cobbler with Oat Topping............................ 113

Coconut Flour Lemon Bars.................................. 114

## Chapter 7: Smoothies ...................................... 115

Green Detox Smoothie........................................ 115

Berry Blast Smoothie......................................... 116

Spinach and Pineapple Smoothie............................ 117

Mango Ginger Smoothie ............................................... 118

Avocado Banana Smoothie ........................................... 119

Kale and Blueberry Smoothie ...................................... 120

Chocolate Protein Smoothie ........................................ 122

Peach Almond Smoothie ............................................. 123

Citrus Burst Smoothie ................................................. 124

Cucumber Mint Smoothie ........................................... 125

Tropical Turmeric Smoothie ....................................... 126

Raspberry Coconut Smoothie ..................................... 127

Coffee and Almond Butter Smoothie ......................... 128

Carrot Cake Smoothie ................................................ 129

Mixed Berry Protein Smoothie ................................... 131

**CONCLUSION** ................................................................ **133**

# INTRODUCTION

I n today's world, Type 2 Diabetes has become increasingly prevalent, affecting millions of people globally. Understanding this condition, along with the importance of diet and meal planning, is crucial for managing blood sugar levels and living a healthy and fulfilling life.

## Understanding Type 2 Diabetes:

Type 2 Diabetes is a chronic condition where your body either doesn't produce enough insulin, or it doesn't use insulin effectively. Insulin is a hormone responsible for transferring glucose, or sugar, from your bloodstream to your cells for energy. This inadequate utilization leads to blood sugar levels rising above normal, causing various health complications.

**Symptoms of Type 2 Diabetes:**

- Frequent urination

- Excessive thirst
- Increased hunger
- Unexplained weight loss
- Fatigue
- Blurred vision
- Slow-healing sores

## Importance of a Healthy Diet:

For individuals with Type 2 Diabetes, a healthy diet plays a pivotal role in managing blood sugar levels. Eating the right foods can:

1. **Reduce blood sugar spikes**: Choose whole grains, fruits, vegetables, and lean proteins over sugary drinks, processed foods, and unhealthy fats.
2. **Improve insulin sensitivity**: This allows your body to use insulin more effectively, resulting in better blood sugar control.
3. **Promote weight loss**: Maintaining a healthy weight can significantly improve diabetes management.
4. **Reduce the risk of complications**: A healthy diet can help prevent various diabetes-related

complications like heart disease, stroke, and nerve damage.

## Basics of Meal Planning for Diabetes:

Here are some key principles for meal planning with Type 2 Diabetes:

1.  **Consistency**: Aim to eat three regular meals and two to three healthy snacks daily. This helps regulate blood sugar levels and prevents spikes.
2.  **Portion Control**: Pay attention to portion sizes. Using measuring cups and spoons can help ensure you're eating the recommended amounts.
3.  **Carbohydrate Counting**: Learn to count carbohydrates in your meals. Carbohydrates have the biggest impact on blood sugar levels, so monitoring your intake is crucial.
4.  **Choose Nutrient-Dense Foods**: Focus on whole grains, fruits, vegetables, lean proteins, and healthy

fats. These foods provide essential nutrients and keep you feeling full.

5. **Limit Added Sugars and Unhealthy Fats**: Avoid sugary drinks, processed foods, and unhealthy fats like saturated and trans fats. These can contribute to blood sugar spikes and weight gain.

6. **Read Food Labels**: Pay close attention to food labels to understand the carbohydrate content and other nutritional information.

7. **Stay Hydrated**: Drink plenty of water throughout the day to prevent dehydration and promote overall health.

Remember, managing Type 2 Diabetes is a journey, and a healthy diet is your compass. By incorporating these principles and consulting with your healthcare team, you can take control of your health and live a well-balanced and fulfilling life.

## Week 1:

Day 1:

- Breakfast: Quinoa Breakfast Bowl
- Lunch: Grilled Chicken Salad
- Dinner: Baked Chicken Breast with Roasted Vegetables
- Snacks: Guacamole with Veggie Sticks
- Dessert: Berry and Yogurt Parfait

Day 2:

- Breakfast: Vegetable Omelette
- Lunch: Quinoa and Black Bean Bowl
- Dinner: Quinoa-Stuffed Bell Peppers
- Snacks: Greek Yogurt Dip with Cucumber Slices
- Dessert: Dark Chocolate-Dipped Strawberries

Day 3:

- Breakfast: Greek Yogurt Parfait
- Lunch: Turkey and Veggie Wrap

- Dinner: Salmon with Lemon-Dill Sauce

- Snacks: Mixed Nuts and Seeds

- Dessert: Baked Apples with Cinnamon

Day 4:

- Breakfast: Chia Seed Pudding

- Lunch: Lentil Soup

- Dinner: Eggplant and Tomato Gratin

- Snacks: Cheese and Whole Grain Crackers

- Dessert: Sugar-Free Pumpkin Pie

Day 5:

- Breakfast: Whole Grain Pancakes

- Lunch: Shrimp and Broccoli Stir-Fry

- Dinner: Turkey and Sweet Potato Casserole

- Snacks: Hummus and Carrot Sticks

- Dessert: Greek Yogurt Popsicles

Day 6:

- Breakfast: Avocado Toast with Poached Egg

- Lunch: Chickpea and Vegetable Curry

- Dinner: Stir-Fried Tofu with Broccoli

- Snacks: Cottage Cheese and Pineapple
- Dessert: Almond Flour Chocolate Chip Cookies

Day 7:

- Breakfast: Berry and Almond Smoothie Bowl
- Lunch: Turkey and Avocado Lettuce Wraps
- Dinner: Spaghetti Squash with Marinara Sauce
- Snacks: Edamame with Sea Salt
- Dessert: Chia Seed Chocolate Pudding

## Week 2:

Day 8:

- Breakfast: Spinach and Feta Breakfast Wrap
- Lunch: Caprese Salad with Balsamic Glaze
- Dinner: Teriyaki Chicken Skillet
- Snacks: Roasted Chickpeas
- Dessert: Fresh Fruit Salad

Day 9:

- Breakfast: Overnight Oats with Berries
- Lunch: Grilled Salmon with Asparagus
- Dinner: Cod with Mediterranean Salsa

- Snacks: Avocado and Tomato Salsa
- Dessert: Avocado Chocolate Mousse

Day 10:

- Breakfast: Sweet Potato Hash with Turkey Sausage
- Lunch: Zucchini Noodles with Pesto
- Dinner: Mushroom and Spinach Stuffed Chicken
- Snacks: Apple Slices with Almond Butter
- Dessert: Banana Walnut Muffins

Day 11:

- Breakfast: Egg and Veggie Muffins
- Lunch: Chicken and Vegetable Skewers
- Dinner: Beef and Vegetable Stir-Fry
- Snacks: Veggie Spring Rolls
- Dessert: Ricotta and Berry Tartlets

Day 12:

- Breakfast: Cottage Cheese and Fruit Plate
- Lunch: Spinach and Mushroom Quesadilla
- Dinner: Baked Cod with Lemon and Herbs
- Snacks: Kale Chips

* Dessert: Mango Sorbet

Day 13:

* Breakfast: Almond Butter and Banana Toast
* Lunch: Tomato Basil Soup
* Dinner: Butternut Squash and Lentil Curry
* Snacks: Mozzarella and Tomato Skewers
* Dessert: Pistachio Date Balls

Day 14:

* Breakfast: Veggie and Cheese Breakfast Quesadilla
* Lunch: Cauliflower Fried Rice
* Dinner: Grilled Veggie and Hummus Wrap
* Snacks: Trail Mix with Dried Fruits
* Dessert: Peach Cobbler with Oat Topping

## Week 3:

Day 15:

* Breakfast: Smoked Salmon and Cream Cheese Bagel
* Lunch: Tuna Salad Lettuce Wraps
* Dinner: Baked Pork Chops with Apple Compote
* Snacks: Sweet Potato Fries with Yogurt Dip

- Dessert: Coconut Flour Lemon Bars

Day 16:

- Breakfast: Quinoa Breakfast Bowl
- Lunch: Grilled Chicken Salad
- Dinner: Baked Chicken Breast with Roasted Vegetables
- Snacks: Guacamole with Veggie Sticks
- Dessert: Berry and Yogurt Parfait

Day 17:

- Breakfast: Vegetable Omelette
- Lunch: Quinoa and Black Bean Bowl
- Dinner: Quinoa-Stuffed Bell Peppers
- Snacks: Greek Yogurt Dip with Cucumber Slices
- Dessert: Dark Chocolate-Dipped Strawberries

Day 18:

- Breakfast: Greek Yogurt Parfait
- Lunch: Turkey and Veggie Wrap
- Dinner: Salmon with Lemon-Dill Sauce
- Snacks: Mixed Nuts and Seeds

- Dessert: Baked Apples with Cinnamon

Day 19:

- Breakfast: Chia Seed Pudding
- Lunch: Lentil Soup
- Dinner: Eggplant and Tomato Gratin
- Snacks: Cheese and Whole Grain Crackers
- Dessert: Sugar-Free Pumpkin Pie

Day 20:

- Breakfast: Whole Grain Pancakes
- Lunch: Shrimp and Broccoli Stir-Fry
- Dinner: Turkey and Sweet Potato Casserole
- Snacks: Hummus and Carrot Sticks
- Dessert: Greek Yogurt Popsicles

Day 21:

- Breakfast: Avocado Toast with Poached Egg
- Lunch: Chickpea and Vegetable Curry
- Dinner: Stir-Fried Tofu with Broccoli
- Snacks: Cottage Cheese and Pineapple
- Dessert: Almond Flour Chocolate Chip Cookies

Day 22:

- Breakfast: Berry and Almond Smoothie Bowl
- Lunch: Turkey and Avocado Lettuce Wraps
- Dinner: Spaghetti Squash with Marinara Sauce
- Snacks: Edamame with Sea Salt
- Dessert: Chia Seed Chocolate Pudding

Day 23:

- Breakfast: Spinach and Feta Breakfast Wrap
- Lunch: Caprese Salad with Balsamic Glaze
- Dinner: Teriyaki Chicken Skillet
- Snacks: Roasted Chickpeas
- Dessert: Fresh Fruit Salad

Day 24:

- Breakfast: Overnight Oats with Berries
- Lunch: Grilled Salmon with Asparagus
- Dinner: Cod with Mediterranean Salsa
- Snacks: Avocado and Tomato Salsa
- Dessert: Avocado Chocolate Mousse

Day 25:

- Breakfast: Sweet Potato Hash with Turkey Sausage
- Lunch: Zucchini Noodles with Pesto
- Dinner: Mushroom and Spinach Stuffed Chicken
- Snacks: Apple Slices with Almond Butter
- Dessert: Banana Walnut Muffins

Day 26:

- Breakfast: Egg and Veggie Muffins
- Lunch: Chicken and Vegetable Skewers
- Dinner: Beef and Vegetable Stir-Fry
- Snacks: Veggie Spring Rolls
- Dessert: Ricotta and Berry Tartlets

Day 27:

- Breakfast: Cottage Cheese and Fruit Plate
- Lunch: Spinach and Mushroom Quesadilla
- Dinner: Baked Cod with Lemon and Herbs
- Snacks: Kale Chips
- Dessert: Mango Sorbet

Day 28:

- Breakfast: Almond Butter and Banana Toast
- Lunch: Tomato Basil Soup
- Dinner: Butternut Squash and Lentil Curry
- Snacks: Mozzarella and Tomato Skewers
- Dessert: Pistachio Date Balls

Day 29:

- Breakfast: Veggie and Cheese Breakfast Quesadilla
- Lunch: Cauliflower Fried Rice
- Dinner: Grilled Veggie and Hummus Wrap
- Snacks: Trail Mix with Dried Fruits
- Dessert: Peach Cobbler with Oat Topping

Day 30:

- Breakfast: Smoked Salmon and Cream Cheese Bagel
- Lunch: Tuna Salad Lettuce Wraps
- Dinner: Baked Pork Chops with Apple Compote
- Snacks: Sweet Potato Fries with Yogurt Dip
- Dessert: Coconut Flour Lemon Bars

Feel free to adjust the plan based on personal preferences and dietary needs. Remember to stay mindful of portion sizes.

# Chapter 2: Breakfast Recipes

Welcome to Chapter 2 of our "Type 2 Diabetes Cookbook for Beginners," where we embark on a delicious journey through 15 wholesome breakfast recipes tailored for your well-being. Each recipe is thoughtfully crafted to not only satisfy your taste buds but also support your nutritional needs.

## Quinoa Breakfast Bowl

Ingredients:

- 1/2 cup quinoa, rinsed
- 1 cup almond milk
- 1/2 cup mixed berries
- 1 tablespoon chopped nuts
- 1 teaspoon honey

Instructions:

1. Cook quinoa according to package instructions using almond milk.

2. Top with mixed berries, chopped nuts, and a drizzle
   of honey.

3. Enjoy!

Nutrition Information:

- Calories: 300

- Protein: 10g

- Carbohydrates: 45g

- Fat: 8g

- Fiber: 7g

- Sugar: 8g

- Portion Size: 1 bowl

## Vegetable Omelette

Ingredients:

- 2 eggs

- 1/4 cup diced bell peppers

- 1/4 cup diced tomatoes

- 1/4 cup spinach

- Salt and pepper to taste

Instructions:

1. Whisk eggs in a bowl and season with salt and pepper.
2. Pour the mixture into a heated non-stick pan.
3. Add bell peppers, tomatoes, and spinach.
4. Cook until the eggs are set, then fold in half.
5. Serve hot.

Nutrition Information:

- Calories: 200
- Protein: 14g
- Carbohydrates: 6g
- Fat: 14g
- Fiber: 2g
- Sugar: 3g
- Portion Size: 1 omelette

## Greek Yogurt Parfait

Ingredients:

- 1 cup Greek yogurt
- 1/2 cup granola
- 1/2 cup mixed berries

- 1 tablespoon honey

Instructions:

1. In a glass, layer Greek yogurt, granola, and mixed berries.
2. Repeat the layers.
3. Drizzle with honey.

Nutrition Information:

- Calories: 350
- Protein: 20g
- Carbohydrates: 45g
- Fat: 12g
- Fiber: 6g
- Sugar: 18g
- Portion Size: 1 parfait

## Chia Seed Pudding

Ingredients:

- 2 tablespoons chia seeds
- 1 cup almond milk
- 1/2 teaspoon vanilla extract

- 1 tablespoon maple syrup
- Fresh fruit for topping

Instructions:

1. Mix chia seeds, almond milk, vanilla extract, and maple syrup.
2. Refrigerate overnight.
3. Top with fresh fruit before serving.

Nutrition Information:

- Calories: 180
- Protein: 5g
- Carbohydrates: 20g
- Fat: 9g
- Fiber: 7g
- Sugar: 8g
- Portion Size: 1 serving

## Whole Grain Pancakes

Ingredients:

- 1 cup whole grain pancake mix
- 1 cup almond milk

- 1 teaspoon cinnamon
- Fresh berries for topping

Instructions:

1. Mix pancake mix, almond milk, and cinnamon until smooth.
2. Cook pancakes on a griddle until golden brown.
3. Top with fresh berries.

Nutrition Information:

- Calories: 250
- Protein: 8g
- Carbohydrates: 40g
- Fat: 6g
- Fiber: 5g
- Sugar: 5g
- Portion Size: 2 pancakes

## Avocado Toast with Poached Egg

Ingredients:

- 1 slice whole grain bread
- 1/2 avocado, mashed

- 1 poached egg
- Salt and pepper to taste

Instructions:

1. Toast the bread and spread mashed avocado.
2. Top with a poached egg.
3. Season with salt and pepper.

Nutrition Information:

- Calories: 220
- Protein: 10g
- Carbohydrates: 20g
- Fat: 12g
- Fiber: 7g
- Sugar: 1g
- Portion Size: 1 serving

## Berry and Almond Smoothie Bowl

Ingredients:

- 1 cup mixed berries
- 1/2 banana
- 1/2 cup almond milk

- 1 tablespoon almond butter
- Toppings: sliced almonds, chia seeds

Instructions:

1. Blend berries, banana, almond milk, and almond butter.
2. Pour into a bowl and add toppings.

Nutrition Information:

- Calories: 280
- Protein: 8g
- Carbohydrates: 35g
- Fat: 14g
- Fiber: 9g
- Sugar: 15g
- Portion Size: 1 bowl

## Spinach and Feta Breakfast Wrap

Ingredients:

- 1 whole wheat tortilla
- 2 eggs, scrambled
- Handful of fresh spinach

- 2 tablespoons feta cheese
- Salsa for topping

Instructions:

1. Fill the tortilla with scrambled eggs, spinach, and feta.
2. Roll into a wrap and top with salsa.

Nutrition Information:

- Calories: 300
- Protein: 15g
- Carbohydrates: 25g
- Fat: 16g
- Fiber: 5g
- Sugar: 3g
- Portion Size: 1 wrap

## Overnight Oats with Berries

Ingredients:

- 1/2 cup rolled oats
- 1/2 cup almond milk
- 1/2 cup mixed berries

- 1 tablespoon chia seeds

- 1 teaspoon honey

Instructions:

1.  Mix oats, almond milk, berries, and chia seeds.

2.  Refrigerate overnight.

3.  Drizzle with honey before serving.

Nutrition Information:

- Calories: 220

- Protein: 8g

- Carbohydrates: 35g

- Fat: 6g

- Fiber: 8g

- Sugar: 8g

- Portion Size: 1 serving

## Sweet Potato Hash with Turkey Sausage

Ingredients:

- 1 sweet potato, diced

- 1/2 cup lean turkey sausage, crumbled
- 1/4 cup red bell pepper, diced
- 1/4 cup onion, diced
- 1 tablespoon olive oil

Instructions:

1. Sauté sweet potato, turkey sausage, bell pepper, and onion in olive oil until cooked.
2. Serve hot.

Nutrition Information:

- Calories: 280
- Protein: 12g
- Carbohydrates: 30g
- Fat: 14g
- Fiber: 6g
- Sugar: 8g
- Portion Size: 1 serving

## Egg and Veggie Muffins

Ingredients:

- 4 eggs

- 1/2 cup diced vegetables (bell peppers, spinach, tomatoes)
- Salt and pepper to taste
- 1/4 cup shredded cheese (optional)

Instructions:

1. Preheat oven to 350°F (175°C).
2. In a bowl, whisk eggs and add diced vegetables.
3. Season with salt and pepper.
4. Pour into muffin cups and bake for 15-20 minutes.
5. Optional: Sprinkle shredded cheese on top.

Nutrition Information:

- Calories: 180
- Protein: 12g
- Carbohydrates: 4g
- Fat: 12g
- Fiber: 2g
- Sugar: 2g
- Portion Size: 2 muffins

# Cottage Cheese and Fruit Plate

Ingredients:

- 1/2 cup low-fat cottage cheese
- 1/2 cup mixed fruit (berries, melon, grapes)
- 1 tablespoon chopped nuts
- 1 teaspoon honey

Instructions:

1. Arrange cottage cheese on a plate.
2. Top with mixed fruit, chopped nuts, and a drizzle of honey.

Nutrition Information:

- Calories: 200
- Protein: 10g
- Carbohydrates: 20g
- Fat: 8g
- Fiber: 4g
- Sugar: 12g
- Portion Size: 1 serving

# Almond Butter and Banana Toast

Ingredients:

- 1 slice whole grain bread
- 1 tablespoon almond butter
- 1/2 banana, sliced
- Cinnamon for topping

Instructions:

1. Toast the bread and spread almond butter.
2. Top with banana slices and a sprinkle of cinnamon.

Nutrition Information:

- Calories: 250
- Protein: 8g
- Carbohydrates: 30g
- Fat: 12g
- Fiber: 6g
- Sugar: 10g
- Portion Size: 1 serving

# Veggie and Cheese Breakfast Quesadilla

Ingredients:

- 1 whole wheat tortilla
- 1/2 cup egg whites
- 1/4 cup diced bell peppers
- 1/4 cup diced tomatoes
- 1/4 cup shredded cheese

Instructions:

1. In a pan, cook egg whites with bell peppers and tomatoes.
2. Place the cooked mixture on half of the tortilla.
3. Sprinkle shredded cheese and fold the tortilla in half.
4. Cook until the cheese melts.

Nutrition Information:

- Calories: 280
- Protein: 18g
- Carbohydrates: 25g
- Fat: 12g
- Fiber: 5g

- Sugar: 3g

- Portion Size: 1 quesadilla

# Smoked Salmon and Cream Cheese Bagel

Ingredients:

- 1 whole grain bagel, toasted

- 2 tablespoons cream cheese

- 2 ounces smoked salmon

- Sliced cucumber and capers for topping

Instructions:

1. Spread cream cheese on the toasted bagel.

2. Top with smoked salmon, sliced cucumber, and capers.

Nutrition Information:

- Calories: 320

- Protein: 20g

- Carbohydrates: 35g

- Fat: 12g

- Fiber: 5g
- Sugar: 2g
- Portion Size: 1 bagel

# Chapter 3: Lunch Recipes

These carefully crafted recipes not only prioritize health but also bring a burst of flavors to your midday meals. Each dish is thoughtfully designed to provide essential nutrients, balanced proportions, and a delightful culinary experience. Let's embark on a journey of tasty and diabetes-friendly lunch options.

## Grilled Chicken Salad

Ingredients:

- 2 boneless, skinless chicken breasts
- 4 cups mixed salad greens
- 1 cup cherry tomatoes, halved
- 1 cucumber, sliced
- 1/4 cup feta cheese, crumbled
- 2 tablespoons olive oil
- 1 tablespoon balsamic vinegar
- Salt and pepper to taste

Instructions:

1. Season chicken breasts with salt and pepper, then grill until fully cooked.
2. In a large bowl, combine salad greens, cherry tomatoes, cucumber, and feta cheese.
3. Slice grilled chicken and place on top of the salad.
4. Whisk together olive oil and balsamic vinegar, drizzle over the salad.
5. Toss gently and serve.

Nutrition Information (per serving):

- Calories: 350
- Protein: 30g
- Carbohydrates: 12g
- Fat: 18g
- Fiber: 4g
- Sugar: 5g
- Portion Size: 1 serving

## Quinoa and Black Bean Bowl

Ingredients:

- 1 cup cooked quinoa

- 1 cup black beans, drained and rinsed
- 1 cup corn kernels
- 1 bell pepper, diced
- 1/4 cup fresh cilantro, chopped
- 2 tablespoons lime juice
- 1 tablespoon olive oil
- Salt and cumin to taste

Instructions:

1. In a bowl, combine cooked quinoa, black beans, corn, bell pepper, and cilantro.
2. In a small bowl, whisk together lime juice, olive oil, salt, and cumin.
3. Pour the dressing over the quinoa mixture and toss until well combined.
4. Serve at room temperature or chilled.

Nutrition Information (per serving):

- Calories: 280
- Protein: 10g
- Carbohydrates: 45g
- Fat: 6g

- Fiber: 8g

- Sugar: 2g

- Portion Size: 1 serving


## Turkey and Veggie Wrap

Ingredients:

- 4 whole-grain tortillas

- 1 pound lean ground turkey

- 1 cup mixed vegetables (bell peppers, onions, zucchini)

- 1 teaspoon olive oil

- 1 teaspoon taco seasoning

- 1/2 cup salsa

- 1/4 cup Greek yogurt (optional)


Instructions:

1. In a skillet, heat olive oil and sauté mixed vegetables until tender.

2. Add ground turkey and taco seasoning, cook until turkey is browned.

3. Warm tortillas and spoon turkey mixture onto each.

4. Top with salsa and a dollop of Greek yogurt if desired.

5. Roll up and enjoy.

Nutrition Information (per serving):

- Calories: 320
- Protein: 25g
- Carbohydrates: 30g
- Fat: 12g
- Fiber: 6g
- Sugar: 5g
- Portion Size: 1 wrap

## Lentil Soup

Ingredients:

- 1 cup dried green lentils, rinsed
- 1 onion, diced
- 2 carrots, diced
- 2 celery stalks, chopped
- 3 cloves garlic, minced
- 1 can (14 oz) diced tomatoes
- 6 cups vegetable broth

- 1 teaspoon cumin
- 1 teaspoon smoked paprika
- Salt and pepper to taste
- Fresh parsley for garnish

Instructions:

1. In a large pot, sauté onions, carrots, celery, and garlic until softened.
2. Add lentils, diced tomatoes, vegetable broth, cumin, smoked paprika, salt, and pepper.
3. Bring to a boil, then reduce heat and simmer for 25-30 minutes or until lentils are tender.
4. Garnish with fresh parsley before serving.

Nutrition Information (per serving):

- Calories: 220
- Protein: 14g
- Carbohydrates: 40g
- Fat: 1g
- Fiber: 15g
- Sugar: 6g
- Portion Size: 1 cup

# Shrimp and Broccoli Stir-Fry

Ingredients:

- 1 pound shrimp, peeled and deveined
- 2 cups broccoli florets
- 1 bell pepper, sliced
- 2 tablespoons low-sodium soy sauce
- 1 tablespoon hoisin sauce
- 1 tablespoon sesame oil
- 2 cloves garlic, minced
- 1 teaspoon ginger, grated
- 2 green onions, sliced

Instructions:

1. In a wok or skillet, heat sesame oil and sauté garlic and ginger.
2. Add shrimp and stir-fry until pink and opaque.
3. Add broccoli and bell pepper, continue stir-frying until vegetables are tender-crisp.
4. Mix in soy sauce and hoisin sauce, stir to coat.
5. Garnish with green onions and serve over brown rice.

Nutrition Information (per serving):

- Calories: 280

- Protein: 30g

- Carbohydrates: 15g

- Fat: 10g

- Fiber: 5g

- Sugar: 4g

- Portion Size: 1 cup

## Chickpea and Vegetable Curry

Ingredients:

- 1 can (15 oz) chickpeas, drained and rinsed

- 1 eggplant, diced

- 1 bell pepper, chopped

- 1 onion, diced

- 2 cloves garlic, minced

- 1 can (14 oz) coconut milk

- 2 tablespoons curry powder

- 1 teaspoon turmeric

- Salt and pepper to taste

- Fresh cilantro for garnish

Instructions:

1. In a pot, sauté onions and garlic until fragrant.
2. Add eggplant and bell pepper, cook until softened.
3. Stir in chickpeas, curry powder, turmeric, salt, and pepper.
4. Pour in coconut milk and simmer until the curry thickens.
5. Garnish with fresh cilantro before serving.

Nutrition Information (per serving):

- Calories: 340
- Protein: 10g
- Carbohydrates: 30g
- Fat: 20g
- Fiber: 8g
- Sugar: 8g
- Portion Size: 1 cup

## Turkey and Avocado Lettuce Wraps

Ingredients:

- 1 pound ground turkey
- 1 tablespoon olive oil

- 1 teaspoon chili powder
- 1/2 teaspoon cumin
- 1/2 teaspoon garlic powder
- Salt and pepper to taste
- Lettuce leaves (such as iceberg or butter lettuce)
- 1 avocado, sliced
- Salsa for topping

Instructions:

1. In a skillet, heat olive oil and cook ground turkey until browned.
2. Season with chili powder, cumin, garlic powder, salt, and pepper.
3. Spoon the turkey mixture onto lettuce leaves.
4. Top with sliced avocado and salsa.
5. Wrap and enjoy.

Nutrition Information (per serving):

- Calories: 290
- Protein: 25g
- Carbohydrates: 8g
- Fat: 18g

- Fiber: 5g
- Sugar: 2g
- Portion Size: 2 wraps

## Caprese Salad with Balsamic Glaze

Ingredients:

- 2 large tomatoes, sliced
- 1 ball fresh mozzarella, sliced
- Fresh basil leaves
- 2 tablespoons balsamic glaze
- Salt and pepper to taste

Instructions:

1. Arrange tomato and mozzarella slices on a serving plate.
2. Tuck fresh basil leaves between the tomato and mozzarella slices.
3. Drizzle balsamic glaze over the salad.
4. Sprinkle with salt and pepper to taste.
5. Serve immediately.

Nutrition Information (per serving):

- Calories: 180
- Protein: 10g
- Carbohydrates: 10g
- Fat: 12g
- Fiber: 2g
- Sugar: 5g
- Portion Size: 1 serving

## Grilled Salmon with Asparagus

Ingredients:

- 4 salmon fillets
- 1 bunch asparagus, trimmed
- 2 tablespoons olive oil
- 1 lemon, sliced
- 2 teaspoons dill, chopped
- Salt and pepper to taste

Instructions:

1. Preheat grill to medium-high heat.
2. Brush salmon fillets and asparagus with olive oil.
3. Season with salt, pepper, and chopped dill.

4.  Grill salmon for 4-5 minutes per side or until cooked through.

5.  Grill asparagus until tender-crisp.

6.  Serve with lemon slices.

Nutrition Information (per serving):

- Calories: 320

- Protein: 30g

- Carbohydrates: 6g

- Fat: 20g

- Fiber: 3g

- Sugar: 2g

- Portion Size: 1 fillet with asparagus

## Zucchini Noodles with Pesto

Ingredients:

- 4 medium-sized zucchini, spiralized

- 1 cup cherry tomatoes, halved

- 1/2 cup pine nuts, toasted

- 1/2 cup fresh basil leaves

- 1/4 cup Parmesan cheese, grated

- 2 cloves garlic, minced

- 1/2 cup olive oil
- Salt and pepper to taste

Instructions:

1. In a blender, combine basil, pine nuts, Parmesan, and garlic.
2. With the blender running, slowly add olive oil until a smooth pesto forms.
3. In a large bowl, toss zucchini noodles with cherry tomatoes and pesto.
4. Season with salt and pepper.
5. Serve chilled or at room temperature.

Nutrition Information (per serving):

- Calories: 280
- Protein: 5g
- Carbohydrates: 10g
- Fat: 25g
- Fiber: 3g
- Sugar: 5g
- Portion Size: 1 serving

# Chicken and Vegetable Skewers

Ingredients:

- 1 pound boneless, skinless chicken breast, cut into cubes
- 2 bell peppers, cut into chunks
- 1 red onion, cut into wedges
- 1 zucchini, sliced
- 2 tablespoons olive oil
- 1 teaspoon Italian seasoning
- Salt and pepper to taste

Instructions:

1. Preheat grill to medium-high heat.
2. Thread chicken, bell peppers, red onion, and zucchini onto skewers.
3. In a bowl, whisk together olive oil, Italian seasoning, salt, and pepper.
4. Brush skewers with the olive oil mixture.
5. Grill for 10-12 minutes, turning occasionally, until chicken is cooked through.

Nutrition Information (per serving):

- Calories: 280
- Protein: 25g
- Carbohydrates: 10g
- Fat: 15g
- Fiber: 3g
- Sugar: 6g
- Portion Size: 2 skewers

## Spinach and Mushroom Quesadilla

Ingredients:

- 4 whole-grain tortillas
- 2 cups fresh spinach leaves
- 1 cup mushrooms, sliced
- 1 cup shredded mozzarella cheese
- 1 tablespoon olive oil
- 1 teaspoon garlic powder
- Salt and pepper to taste

Instructions:

1. In a skillet, heat olive oil and sauté mushrooms until golden brown.

2. Add spinach and cook until wilted.

3. Season with garlic powder, salt, and pepper.

4. On a tortilla, layer spinach and mushroom mixture with mozzarella.

5. Top with another tortilla and cook on a griddle until cheese is melted and tortilla is crispy.

Nutrition Information (per serving):

- Calories: 290
- Protein: 15g
- Carbohydrates: 30g
- Fat: 12g
- Fiber: 5g
- Sugar: 3g
- Portion Size: 1 quesadilla

## Tomato Basil Soup

Ingredients:

- 6 large tomatoes, chopped
- 1 onion, diced
- 3 cloves garlic, minced
- 4 cups vegetable broth

- 1/2 cup fresh basil leaves, chopped

- 1 teaspoon olive oil

- Salt and pepper to taste

- Greek yogurt for garnish (optional)

Instructions:

1. In a pot, sauté onions and garlic in olive oil until softened.

2. Add chopped tomatoes and cook until they release their juices.

3. Pour in vegetable broth and bring to a simmer.

4. Add fresh basil and season with salt and pepper.

5. Blend the soup until smooth. Serve with a dollop of Greek yogurt if desired.

Nutrition Information (per serving):

- Calories: 120

- Protein: 3g

- Carbohydrates: 20g

- Fat: 4g

- Fiber: 5g

- Sugar: 12g

- Portion Size: 1 cup

## Cauliflower Fried Rice

Ingredients:

- 1 head cauliflower, grated
- 1 cup mixed vegetables (peas, carrots, corn)
- 2 eggs, beaten
- 3 green onions, sliced
- 2 tablespoons soy sauce
- 1 tablespoon sesame oil
- 1 teaspoon ginger, minced
- 1 teaspoon garlic, minced

Instructions:

1. In a large skillet, heat sesame oil and sauté ginger and garlic.
2. Add grated cauliflower and mixed vegetables, stir-fry until tender.
3. Push the cauliflower mixture to the side, pour beaten eggs into the skillet.
4. Scramble the eggs and mix with the cauliflower.

5. Stir in soy sauce and green onions. Cook until heated through.

Nutrition Information (per serving):

- Calories: 180
- Protein: 10g
- Carbohydrates: 15g
- Fat: 9g
- Fiber: 6g
- Sugar: 6g
- Portion Size: 1 cup

## Tuna Salad Lettuce Wraps

Ingredients:

- 2 cans (5 oz each) tuna, drained
- 1/2 cup celery, diced
- 1/4 cup red onion, finely chopped
- 2 tablespoons mayonnaise
- 1 tablespoon Dijon mustard
- Salt and pepper to taste
- Lettuce leaves for wrapping

Instructions:

1.  In a bowl, mix tuna, celery, red onion, mayonnaise, and Dijon mustard.
2.  Season with salt and pepper to taste.
3.  Spoon the tuna salad onto lettuce leaves.
4.  Wrap and secure with toothpicks if needed.
5.  Serve chilled.

Nutrition Information (per serving):

- Calories: 220
- Protein: 20g
- Carbohydrates: 5g
- Fat: 15g
- Fiber: 2g
- Sugar: 2g
- Portion Size: 2 wraps

# Chapter 4: Dinner Recipes

Each recipe not only tantalizes your taste buds but also adheres to the principles of managing type 2 diabetes. From succulent Baked Chicken Breast with Roasted Vegetables to the flavorful Grilled Veggie and Hummus Wrap, these dishes are a perfect blend of nutrition and deliciousness.

## Baked Chicken Breast with Roasted Vegetables

Ingredients:

- 4 boneless, skinless chicken breasts
- 2 cups mixed vegetables (bell peppers, zucchini, cherry tomatoes)
- 2 tablespoons olive oil
- 1 teaspoon garlic powder
- 1 teaspoon dried thyme
- Salt and pepper to taste

Instructions:

1. Preheat the oven to 400°F (200°C).

2. Place chicken breasts on a baking sheet, surrounded by mixed vegetables.

3. Drizzle olive oil over chicken and vegetables. Sprinkle garlic powder, thyme, salt, and pepper.

4. Bake for 25-30 minutes or until chicken is cooked through.

5. Serve hot, and enjoy!

Nutrition Information (per serving):

- Calories: 300
- Protein: 30g
- Carbohydrates: 15g
- Fat: 12g
- Fiber: 5g
- Sugar: 5g
- Portion Size: 1 chicken breast with vegetables

## Quinoa-Stuffed Bell Peppers

Ingredients:

- 4 bell peppers, halved
- 1 cup quinoa, cooked
- 1 cup black beans, drained and rinsed

- 1 cup corn kernels

- 1 cup diced tomatoes

- 1 teaspoon cumin

- 1 teaspoon chili powder

- Salt and pepper to taste

Instructions:

1. Preheat the oven to 375°F (190°C).
2. In a bowl, mix quinoa, black beans, corn, tomatoes, cumin, chili powder, salt, and pepper.
3. Stuff each bell pepper half with the quinoa mixture.
4. Bake for 25-30 minutes or until peppers are tender.
5. Serve warm.

Nutrition Information (per serving):

- Calories: 250

- Protein: 10g

- Carbohydrates: 45g

- Fat: 3g

- Fiber: 8g

- Sugar: 5g

- Portion Size: 2 stuffed pepper halves

# Salmon with Lemon-Dill Sauce

Ingredients:

- 4 salmon fillets
- 2 tablespoons olive oil
- 2 tablespoons fresh lemon juice
- 1 tablespoon fresh dill, chopped
- 1 teaspoon garlic powder
- Salt and pepper to taste

Instructions:

1. Preheat the oven to 400°F (200°C).
2. Place salmon fillets on a baking sheet.
3. In a bowl, mix olive oil, lemon juice, dill, garlic powder, salt, and pepper.
4. Brush the mixture over salmon fillets.
5. Bake for 15-20 minutes or until salmon flakes easily.
6. Serve with additional lemon wedges.

Nutrition Information (per serving):

- Calories: 350
- Protein: 25g
- Carbohydrates: 1g

- Fat: 25g

- Fiber: 0g

- Sugar: 0g

- Portion Size: 1 salmon fillet

# Eggplant and Tomato Gratin

Ingredients:

- 1 large eggplant, thinly sliced

- 2 cups cherry tomatoes, halved

- 1 cup mozzarella cheese, shredded

- 1/4 cup Parmesan cheese, grated

- 2 tablespoons olive oil

- 1 teaspoon dried oregano

- Salt and pepper to taste

Instructions:

1. Preheat the oven to 375°F (190°C).

2. Arrange eggplant slices in a baking dish.

3. Scatter cherry tomatoes over the eggplant.

4. Drizzle olive oil, sprinkle oregano, salt, and pepper.

5. Top with mozzarella and Parmesan cheese.

6. Bake for 25-30 minutes or until bubbly and golden.

7.  Serve as a satisfying side dish.

Nutrition Information (per serving):

- Calories: 220
- Protein: 10g
- Carbohydrates: 15g
- Fat: 15g
- Fiber: 7g
- Sugar: 8g
- Portion Size: 1 cup

## Turkey and Sweet Potato Casserole

Ingredients:

- 1 lb ground turkey
- 2 sweet potatoes, peeled and diced
- 1 onion, diced
- 2 cloves garlic, minced
- 1 cup spinach, chopped
- 1 cup low-sodium chicken broth
- 1 teaspoon paprika
- Salt and pepper to taste

Instructions:

1. Preheat the oven to 375°F (190°C).
2. In a skillet, brown ground turkey with onions and garlic.
3. Add sweet potatoes, spinach, chicken broth, paprika, salt, and pepper.
4. Transfer the mixture to a casserole dish.
5. Bake for 30-35 minutes or until sweet potatoes are tender.
6. Enjoy a hearty and nutritious meal!

Nutrition Information (per serving):

- Calories: 280
- Protein: 20g
- Carbohydrates: 25g
- Fat: 12g
- Fiber: 5g
- Sugar: 5g
- Portion Size: 1 cup

# Stir-Fried Tofu with Broccoli

Ingredients:

- 1 lb firm tofu, cubed
- 2 cups broccoli florets
- 2 tablespoons soy sauce (low sodium)
- 1 tablespoon sesame oil
- 1 teaspoon ginger, minced
- 1 teaspoon garlic, minced
- 1 tablespoon rice vinegar
- Salt and pepper to taste

Instructions:

1. Press tofu to remove excess water, then stir-fry until golden.
2. Add broccoli, ginger, and garlic to the pan and stir-fry until vegetables are tender-crisp.
3. In a bowl, mix soy sauce, sesame oil, and rice vinegar.
4. Pour the sauce over tofu and broccoli, toss to combine.
5. Season with salt and pepper.
6. Serve over brown rice.

Nutrition Information (per serving):

- Calories: 220
- Protein: 15g
- Carbohydrates: 12g
- Fat: 12g
- Fiber: 4g
- Sugar: 2g
- Portion Size: 1 cup

## Spaghetti Squash with Marinara Sauce

Ingredients:

- 1 large spaghetti squash
- 2 cups marinara sauce (sugar-free)
- 1 tablespoon olive oil
- 1 teaspoon dried basil
- 1 teaspoon dried oregano
- Salt and pepper to taste

Instructions:

1. Preheat the oven to 400°F (200°C).

2. Cut the spaghetti squash in half, remove seeds.

3. Brush squash with olive oil, sprinkle with basil, oregano, salt, and pepper.

4. Roast for 40-45 minutes or until squash is fork-tender.

5. Scrape the squash with a fork to create "spaghetti."

6. Serve with warm marinara sauce.

Nutrition Information (per serving):

- Calories: 180
- Protein: 3g
- Carbohydrates: 30g
- Fat: 7g
- Fiber: 8g
- Sugar: 12g
- Portion Size: 1 cup

## Teriyaki Chicken Skillet

Ingredients:

- 1 lb chicken breast, sliced
- 1 cup broccoli, chopped
- 1 red bell pepper, sliced

- 1/4 cup low-sodium teriyaki sauce

- 2 tablespoons olive oil

- 1 tablespoon sesame seeds (optional)

- Salt and pepper to taste

Instructions:

1. In a skillet, heat olive oil and sauté chicken until browned.
2. Add broccoli and bell pepper, continue cooking until vegetables are tender.
3. Pour teriyaki sauce over the chicken and vegetables.
4. Stir until everything is coated and heated through.
5. Garnish with sesame seeds if desired.
6. Serve over brown rice or cauliflower rice.

Nutrition Information (per serving):

- Calories: 280

- Protein: 25g

- Carbohydrates: 15g

- Fat: 12g

- Fiber: 3g

- Sugar: 8g

- Portion Size: 1 cup

## Cod with Mediterranean Salsa

Ingredients:

- 4 cod fillets
- 1 cup cherry tomatoes, diced
- 1/2 cup Kalamata olives, chopped
- 1/4 cup red onion, finely chopped
- 2 tablespoons fresh basil, chopped
- 2 tablespoons olive oil
- 1 tablespoon balsamic vinegar
- Salt and pepper to taste

Instructions:

1. Preheat the oven to 400°F (200°C).
2. Season cod fillets with salt and pepper, then bake for 15-20 minutes or until flaky.
3. In a bowl, combine cherry tomatoes, olives, red onion, basil, olive oil, and balsamic vinegar.
4. Spoon the Mediterranean salsa over the cod fillets.
5. Serve with a side of steamed vegetables or quinoa.

Nutrition Information (per serving):

- Calories: 250
- Protein: 30g
- Carbohydrates: 8g
- Fat: 12g
- Fiber: 2g
- Sugar: 4g
- Portion Size: 1 cod fillet with salsa

## Mushroom and Spinach Stuffed Chicken

Ingredients:

- 4 boneless, skinless chicken breasts
- 1 cup mushrooms, chopped
- 2 cups fresh spinach
- 1/2 cup feta cheese, crumbled
- 2 tablespoons olive oil
- 1 teaspoon garlic powder
- Salt and pepper to taste

Instructions:

1. Preheat the oven to 375°F (190°C).
2. In a skillet, sauté mushrooms and spinach in olive oil until wilted.
3. Butterfly each chicken breast and stuff with the mushroom and spinach mixture.
4. Sprinkle feta cheese over the stuffed chicken.
5. Place the chicken in a baking dish, sprinkle with garlic powder, salt, and pepper.
6. Bake for 25-30 minutes or until chicken is cooked through.
7. Serve with a side salad.

Nutrition Information (per serving):

- Calories: 320
- Protein: 35g
- Carbohydrates: 5g
- Fat: 18g
- Fiber: 2g
- Sugar: 2g
- Portion Size: 1 stuffed chicken breast

# Beef and Vegetable Stir-Fry

Ingredients:

- 1 lb lean beef strips
- 2 cups broccoli florets
- 1 red bell pepper, sliced
- 1 cup snap peas
- 2 tablespoons low-sodium soy sauce
- 1 tablespoon hoisin sauce
- 1 tablespoon sesame oil
- 1 teaspoon ginger, minced
- 2 cloves garlic, minced
- Salt and pepper to taste

Instructions:

1. In a wok or large skillet, stir-fry beef until browned. Remove from the pan.
2. Stir-fry broccoli, bell pepper, and snap peas until crisp-tender.
3. Add back the cooked beef.
4. In a small bowl, mix soy sauce, hoisin sauce, sesame oil, ginger, and garlic.

5.  Pour the sauce over the beef and vegetables, toss to combine.

6.  Season with salt and pepper.

7.  Serve over brown rice or cauliflower rice.

Nutrition Information (per serving):

- Calories: 300

- Protein: 25g

- Carbohydrates: 15g

- Fat: 15g

- Fiber: 4g

- Sugar: 5g

- Portion Size: 1 cup

## Baked Cod with Lemon and Herbs

Ingredients:

- 4 cod fillets

- 2 tablespoons olive oil

- 2 tablespoons fresh lemon juice

- 1 tablespoon fresh parsley, chopped

- 1 teaspoon dried dill

- 1 teaspoon garlic powder

- Salt and pepper to taste

Instructions:

1. Preheat the oven to 400°F (200°C).
2. Place cod fillets in a baking dish.
3. Drizzle with olive oil and lemon juice.
4. Sprinkle with parsley, dill, garlic powder, salt, and pepper.
5. Bake for 15-20 minutes or until the cod is cooked through and flakes easily.
6. Serve with a side of steamed vegetables or a quinoa salad.

Nutrition Information (per serving):

- Calories: 230
- Protein: 30g
- Carbohydrates: 2g
- Fat: 10g
- Fiber: 0g
- Sugar: 0g
- Portion Size: 1 cod fillet

# Butternut Squash and Lentil Curry

Ingredients:

- 1 cup dry lentils, rinsed
- 2 cups butternut squash, diced
- 1 onion, finely chopped
- 2 cloves garlic, minced
- 1 can (14 oz) coconut milk
- 2 tablespoons curry powder
- 1 teaspoon ground turmeric
- Salt and pepper to taste
- Fresh cilantro for garnish

Instructions:

1. In a pot, combine lentils, butternut squash, onion, garlic, coconut milk, curry powder, and turmeric.
2. Bring to a simmer, then cover and cook for 20-25 minutes or until lentils and squash are tender.
3. Season with salt and pepper.
4. Garnish with fresh cilantro before serving.
5. Enjoy over brown rice or quinoa.

Nutrition Information (per serving):

- Calories: 300
- Protein: 15g
- Carbohydrates: 45g
- Fat: 8g
- Fiber: 15g
- Sugar: 3g
- Portion Size: 1 cup

## Grilled Veggie and Hummus Wrap

Ingredients:

- 4 whole-grain wraps
- 2 cups mixed grilled vegetables (zucchini, bell peppers, eggplant)
- 1 cup cherry tomatoes, halved
- 1 cup hummus
- Fresh basil leaves
- Salt and pepper to taste

Instructions:

1. Spread a generous layer of hummus on each wrap.
2. Layer with grilled vegetables and cherry tomatoes.

3. Season with salt and pepper, and top with fresh basil leaves.

4. Roll the wraps and secure with toothpicks if needed.

5. Slice in half and serve.

Nutrition Information (per serving):

- Calories: 280

- Protein: 10g

- Carbohydrates: 40g

- Fat: 10g

- Fiber: 10g

- Sugar: 5g

- Portion Size: 1 wrap

## Baked Pork Chops with Apple Compote

Ingredients:

- 4 boneless pork chops

- 2 apples, peeled and sliced

- 1 tablespoon honey

- 1 teaspoon cinnamon

- 1/2 teaspoon nutmeg

- 1 tablespoon olive oil

- Salt and pepper to taste

Instructions:

1. Preheat the oven to 375°F (190°C).

2. Season pork chops with salt and pepper.

3. In a skillet, heat olive oil and sear pork chops until browned on both sides.

4. In a bowl, mix apple slices, honey, cinnamon, and nutmeg.

5. Place pork chops in a baking dish, top with the apple mixture.

6. Bake for 25-30 minutes or until pork is cooked through.

7. Serve with a side of steamed broccoli or a green salad.

Nutrition Information (per serving):

- Calories: 320

- Protein: 25g

- Carbohydrates: 20g

- Fat: 15g

- Fiber: 5g

- Sugar: 15g

- Portion Size: 1 pork chop with apple compote

# Chapter 5: Snacks and Appetizers



In Chapter 5, we explore a collection of Snacks and Appetizers that are not only delicious but also suitable for those managing type 2 diabetes. These recipes incorporate a variety of flavors and textures to keep your taste buds satisfied.

## Guacamole with Veggie Sticks

Ingredients:

- 2 ripe avocados
- 1 small onion, finely diced
- 1 tomato, diced
- 1 clove garlic, minced
- 1 lime, juiced
- Salt and pepper to taste
- Assorted veggie sticks (carrots, celery, bell peppers)

Instructions:

1. In a bowl, mash the avocados.

2.  Add diced onion, tomato, minced garlic, lime juice, salt, and pepper.

3.  Mix well until ingredients are combined.

4.  Serve with assorted veggie sticks.

Nutrition Information (per serving):

- Calories: 120

- Protein: 2g

- Carbohydrates: 8g

- Fat: 10g

- Fiber: 5g

- Sugar: 1g

- Portion Size: 1/2 cup guacamole with veggie sticks.

## Greek Yogurt Dip with Cucumber Slices

Ingredients:

- 1 cup Greek yogurt

- 1 tablespoon fresh dill, chopped

- 1 teaspoon lemon juice

- Salt and pepper to taste

- Cucumber slices for dipping

Instructions:

1. In a bowl, mix Greek yogurt, chopped dill, lemon juice, salt, and pepper.
2. Refrigerate for at least 30 minutes.
3. Serve chilled with cucumber slices.

Nutrition Information (per serving):

- Calories: 70
- Protein: 10g
- Carbohydrates: 5g
- Fat: 1g
- Fiber: 0g
- Sugar: 3g
- Portion Size: 1/4 cup dip with cucumber slices.

## Mixed Nuts and Seeds

Ingredients:

- 1/4 cup almonds
- 1/4 cup walnuts
- 2 tablespoons pumpkin seeds

* 2 tablespoons sunflower seeds

Instructions:

1. Mix all nuts and seeds together.
2. Portion into snack-sized servings.

Nutrition Information (per serving):

- Calories: 200
- Protein: 8g
- Carbohydrates: 5g
- Fat: 18g
- Fiber: 3g
- Sugar: 1g
- Portion Size: 1/4 cup mixed nuts and seeds.

## Cheese and Whole Grain Crackers

Ingredients:

- 1 ounce of your favorite cheese (cheddar, mozzarella, or goat cheese)
- Whole grain crackers

Instructions:

1. Slice the cheese into bite-sized pieces.
2. Arrange the cheese alongside whole grain crackers.

Nutrition Information (per serving):

- Calories: 150
- Protein: 8g
- Carbohydrates: 10g
- Fat: 9g
- Fiber: 2g
- Sugar: 0g
- Portion Size: 1 ounce cheese with whole grain crackers.

## Hummus and Carrot Sticks

Ingredients:

- 1 cup hummus
- Fresh carrot sticks

Instructions:

1. Place hummus in a serving bowl.
2. Wash and peel carrots, then cut them into sticks.

3.  Dip carrot sticks into hummus and enjoy.

Nutrition Information (per serving):

- Calories: 120
- Protein: 6g
- Carbohydrates: 14g
- Fat: 5g
- Fiber: 6g
- Sugar: 2g
- Portion Size: 1/4 cup hummus with carrot sticks.

## Cottage Cheese and Pineapple

Ingredients:

- 1/2 cup low-fat cottage cheese
- 1/2 cup fresh pineapple chunks

Instructions:

1.  In a bowl, combine cottage cheese and pineapple chunks.
2.  Mix well and serve chilled.

Nutrition Information (per serving):

- Calories: 120
- Protein: 14g
- Carbohydrates: 16g
- Fat: 2g
- Fiber: 2g
- Sugar: 10g
- Portion Size: 1/2 cup cottage cheese with pineapple.

## Edamame with Sea Salt

Ingredients:

- 1 cup edamame (steamed)
- Sea salt to taste

Instructions:

1. Steam edamame according to package instructions.
2. Sprinkle with sea salt and toss to coat.
3. Serve in a bowl for snacking.

Nutrition Information (per serving):

- Calories: 120
- Protein: 11g

- Carbohydrates: 9g

- Fat: 5g

- Fiber: 4g

- Sugar: 3g

- Portion Size: 1 cup edamame with sea salt.


## Roasted Chickpeas

Ingredients:

- 1 can (15 oz) chickpeas, drained and rinsed

- 1 tablespoon olive oil

- 1 teaspoon smoked paprika

- 1/2 teaspoon cumin

- Salt to taste

Instructions:

1. Preheat the oven to 400°F (200°C).

2. In a bowl, toss chickpeas with olive oil, smoked paprika, cumin, and salt.

3. Spread chickpeas on a baking sheet and roast for 20-25 minutes, or until crispy.

4. Allow to cool before serving.

Nutrition Information (per serving):

- Calories: 150
- Protein: 6g
- Carbohydrates: 22g
- Fat: 5g
- Fiber: 6g
- Sugar: 4g
- Portion Size: 1/2 cup roasted chickpeas.

## Avocado and Tomato Salsa

Ingredients:

- 2 ripe avocados, diced
- 1 cup cherry tomatoes, halved
- 1/4 cup red onion, finely chopped
- 1 jalapeño, seeds removed and finely chopped
- 2 tablespoons fresh cilantro, chopped
- Lime juice to taste
- Salt and pepper to taste

Instructions:

1. In a bowl, combine avocados, cherry tomatoes, red onion, jalapeño, and cilantro.

2. Drizzle with lime juice, and season with salt and pepper.

3. Gently toss ingredients until well combined.

Nutrition Information (per serving):

- Calories: 140
- Protein: 2g
- Carbohydrates: 10g
- Fat: 12g
- Fiber: 6g
- Sugar: 2g
- Portion Size: 1/2 cup avocado and tomato salsa.

## Apple Slices with Almond Butter

Ingredients:

- 2 medium apples, sliced
- 1/4 cup almond butter

Instructions:

1. Arrange apple slices on a plate.

2. Warm almond butter slightly and drizzle over the apple slices.

Nutrition Information (per serving):

- Calories: 180

- Protein: 4g

- Carbohydrates: 25g

- Fat: 8g

- Fiber: 6g

- Sugar: 16g

- Portion Size: 1 medium apple with almond butter.


## Veggie Spring Rolls

Ingredients:

- Rice paper wrappers

- 1 cup shredded cabbage

- 1/2 cup matchstick carrots

- 1/2 cup cucumber, julienned

- Fresh mint leaves

- 1/4 cup hoisin sauce for dipping


Instructions:

1. Soften rice paper wrappers according to package instructions.

2.  Place a small amount of shredded cabbage, carrots, cucumber, and mint leaves on each wrapper.

3.  Roll tightly and serve with hoisin sauce for dipping.

Nutrition Information (per serving):

- Calories: 80

- Protein: 2g

- Carbohydrates: 18g

- Fat: 0g

- Fiber: 3g

- Sugar: 5g

- Portion Size: 2 spring rolls with hoisin sauce.

## Kale Chips

Ingredients:

- 1 bunch kale, stems removed and torn into bite-sized pieces

- 1 tablespoon olive oil

- Salt to taste

Instructions:

1.  Preheat the oven to 350°F (175°C).

2.  In a bowl, toss kale with olive oil and salt.

3.  Spread kale on a baking sheet and bake for 10-15 minutes, or until crisp.

Nutrition Information (per serving):

- Calories: 50
- Protein: 2g
- Carbohydrates: 6g
- Fat: 3g
- Fiber: 1g
- Sugar: 1g
- Portion Size: 1 cup kale chips.

## Mozzarella and Tomato Skewers

Ingredients:

- Fresh mozzarella balls
- Cherry tomatoes
- Fresh basil leaves
- Balsamic glaze for drizzling

Instructions:

1.  Thread mozzarella balls, cherry tomatoes, and basil leaves onto skewers.

2.  Arrange on a serving platter and drizzle with balsamic glaze.

Nutrition Information (per serving):

- Calories: 120
- Protein: 6g
- Carbohydrates: 3g
- Fat: 9g
- Fiber: 1g
- Sugar: 2g
- Portion Size: 3 skewers with balsamic glaze.

## Trail Mix with Dried Fruits

Ingredients:

- 1/2 cup almonds
- 1/2 cup walnuts
- 1/4 cup dried cranberries
- 1/4 cup dried apricots, chopped
- 1/4 cup dark chocolate chips

Instructions:

1. Mix all ingredients in a bowl.
2. Portion into snack-sized servings.

Nutrition Information (per serving):

- Calories: 200
- Protein: 5g
- Carbohydrates: 15g
- Fat: 14g
- Fiber: 3g
- Sugar: 9g
- Portion Size: 1/4 cup trail mix.

## Sweet Potato Fries with Yogurt Dip

Ingredients:

- 2 medium sweet potatoes, cut into fries
- 1 tablespoon olive oil
- 1 teaspoon smoked paprika
- Salt and pepper to taste
- 1/2 cup Greek yogurt
- 1 tablespoon chopped fresh dill

Instructions:

1.  Preheat the oven to 425°F (220°C).

2.  In a bowl, toss sweet potato fries with olive oil, smoked paprika, salt, and pepper.

3.  Spread on a baking sheet and bake for 20-25 minutes, or until crispy.

4.  In a small bowl, mix Greek yogurt and chopped dill for dipping.

Nutrition Information (per serving):

- Calories: 180
- Protein: 6g
- Carbohydrates: 30g
- Fat: 5g
- Fiber: 5g
- Sugar: 6g
- Portion Size: 1 cup sweet potato fries with yogurt dip.

# Chapter 6: Desserts

These treats not only satisfy your sweet cravings but also adhere to the principles of a diabetes-friendly diet. Each recipe is crafted to bring joy to your taste buds without compromising on nutritional value. So, let's explore the sweetness of life, one healthy dessert at a time.

## Berry and Yogurt Parfait

Ingredients:

- 1 cup mixed berries (strawberries, blueberries, raspberries)
- 1 cup low-fat Greek yogurt
- 2 tablespoons chopped nuts (almonds, walnuts)

Instructions:

1. In a glass or bowl, layer mixed berries and Greek yogurt.
2. Repeat the layers, finishing with a sprinkle of chopped nuts on top.
3. Chill for 30 minutes before serving.

Nutrition Information (per serving):

- Calories: 180
- Protein: 12g
- Carbohydrates: 20g
- Fat: 7g
- Fiber: 5g
- Sugar: 12g

## Dark Chocolate-Dipped Strawberries

Ingredients:

- 1 cup dark chocolate (70% cocoa or higher)
- 1 pint fresh strawberries, washed and dried

Instructions:

1. Melt dark chocolate in a heatproof bowl.
2. Dip each strawberry into the melted chocolate, covering half.
3. Place on parchment paper and refrigerate until the chocolate hardens.

Nutrition Information (per serving):

- Calories: 120

- Protein: 2g

- Carbohydrates: 15g

- Fat: 8g

- Fiber: 4g

- Sugar: 8g


## Baked Apples with Cinnamon

Ingredients:

- 4 apples, cored and halved

- 2 tablespoons cinnamon

- 2 tablespoons chopped nuts (pecans, almonds)


Instructions:

1. Preheat the oven to 350°F (175°C).

2. Place apples in a baking dish, sprinkle with cinnamon, and add chopped nuts.

3. Bake for 25-30 minutes until apples are tender.


Nutrition Information (per serving):

- Calories: 140

- Protein: 2g

- Carbohydrates: 30g

- Fat: 4g

- Fiber: 6g

- Sugar: 20g

## Sugar-Free Pumpkin Pie

Ingredients:

- 1 can (15 oz) pumpkin puree

- 1 teaspoon pumpkin pie spice

- 1/4 cup sugar substitute

- 2 large eggs

- 1 cup unsweetened almond milk

Instructions:

1. Preheat the oven to 375°F (190°C).

2. In a bowl, mix pumpkin puree, pumpkin pie spice, sugar substitute, eggs, and almond milk.

3. Pour into a pie crust and bake for 45-50 minutes.

Nutrition Information (per serving):

- Calories: 120

- Protein: 5g

- Carbohydrates: 15g

- Fat: 5g

- Fiber: 4g

- Sugar: 2g

## Greek Yogurt Popsicles

Ingredients:

- 2 cups plain Greek yogurt

- 1 cup mixed berries (strawberries, blueberries)

- 2 tablespoons honey

Instructions:

1. In a blender, mix Greek yogurt, berries, and honey.

2. Pour into popsicle molds and freeze for at least 4 hours.

Nutrition Information (per serving):

- Calories: 100

- Protein: 10g

- Carbohydrates: 15g

- Fat: 1g

- Fiber: 2g

- Sugar: 10g

# Almond Flour Chocolate Chip Cookies

Ingredients:

- 2 cups almond flour
- 1/2 cup sugar substitute
- 1/2 cup dark chocolate chips
- 1/2 cup melted coconut oil
- 1 teaspoon vanilla extract

Instructions:

1. Preheat the oven to 350°F (175°C).
2. In a bowl, mix almond flour, sugar substitute, chocolate chips, coconut oil, and vanilla extract.
3. Form into cookies and bake for 12-15 minutes.

Nutrition Information (per serving):

- Calories: 120
- Protein: 3g
- Carbohydrates: 8g
- Fat: 9g
- Fiber: 2g
- Sugar: 1g

# Chia Seed Chocolate Pudding

Ingredients:

- 1/4 cup chia seeds
- 1 cup unsweetened almond milk
- 2 tablespoons cocoa powder
- 1 tablespoon sugar substitute
- 1/2 teaspoon vanilla extract

Instructions:

1. Mix chia seeds, almond milk, cocoa powder, sugar substitute, and vanilla extract in a jar.
2. Refrigerate for at least 2 hours or overnight.

Nutrition Information (per serving):

- Calories: 90
- Protein: 3g
- Carbohydrates: 10g
- Fat: 5g
- Fiber: 6g
- Sugar: 1g

## Fresh Fruit Salad

Ingredients:

- 2 cups mixed fresh fruits (melon, berries, grapes)
- 1 tablespoon fresh mint, chopped
- 1 tablespoon lime juice

Instructions:

1. Combine mixed fruits, chopped mint, and lime juice in a bowl.
2. Toss gently and refrigerate for 30 minutes before serving.

Nutrition Information (per serving):

- Calories: 70
- Protein: 1g
- Carbohydrates: 18g
- Fat: 0g
- Fiber: 3g
- Sugar: 14g

# Avocado Chocolate Mousse

Ingredients:

- 2 ripe avocados
- 1/4 cup cocoa powder
- 1/4 cup sugar substitute
- 1 teaspoon vanilla extract

Instructions:

1. In a blender, combine avocados, cocoa powder, sugar substitute, and vanilla extract.
2. Blend until smooth and refrigerate for at least 1 hour.

Nutrition Information (per serving):

- Calories: 160
- Protein: 3g
- Carbohydrates: 12g
- Fat: 14g
- Fiber: 7g
- Sugar: 1g

# Banana Walnut Muffins

Ingredients:

- 2 ripe bananas, mashed
- 1/2 cup almond flour
- 1/2 cup chopped walnuts
- 1/4 cup coconut oil
- 2 eggs

Instructions:

1. Preheat the oven to 350°F (175°C).
2. Mix mashed bananas, almond flour, chopped walnuts, coconut oil, and eggs.
3. Pour into muffin cups and bake for 20-25 minutes.

Nutrition Information (per serving):

- Calories: 140
- Protein: 4g
- Carbohydrates: 10g
- Fat: 10g
- Fiber: 3g
- Sugar: 4g

# Ricotta and Berry Tartlets

Ingredients:

- 1 cup ricotta cheese
- 1/2 cup mixed berries (strawberries, blueberries)
- 1 tablespoon honey
- 1 teaspoon lemon zest

Instructions:

1. In a bowl, mix ricotta cheese, mixed berries, honey, and lemon zest.
2. Spoon into tartlet shells and refrigerate for 1 hour.

Nutrition Information (per serving):

- Calories: 130
- Protein: 7g
- Carbohydrates: 10g
- Fat: 7g
- Fiber: 2g
- Sugar: 7g

## Mango Sorbet

Ingredients:

- 2 cups frozen mango chunks
- 1/4 cup lime juice
- 2 tablespoons honey

Instructions:

1. In a blender, combine frozen mango chunks, lime juice, and honey.
2. Blend until smooth and freeze for 2 hours.

Nutrition Information (per serving):

- Calories: 110
- Protein: 1g
- Carbohydrates: 28g
- Fat: 0g
- Fiber: 2g
- Sugar: 24g

# Pistachio Date Balls

Ingredients:

- 1 cup dates, pitted
- 1/2 cup pistachios
- 1/4 cup shredded coconut

Instructions:

1. In a food processor, blend dates and pistachios until a sticky dough forms.
2. Roll into balls and coat with shredded coconut.

Nutrition Information (per serving):

- Calories: 120
- Protein: 2g
- Carbohydrates: 20g
- Fat: 5g
- Fiber: 3g
- Sugar: 15g

# Peach Cobbler with Oat Topping

Ingredients:

- 4 cups sliced peaches
- 1 tablespoon lemon juice
- 1/2 cup oats
- 1/4 cup almond flour
- 2 tablespoons melted butter

Instructions:

1. Preheat the oven to 375°F (190°C).
2. Mix sliced peaches with lemon juice and place in a baking dish.
3. In a bowl, combine oats, almond flour, and melted butter. Sprinkle over peaches.
4. Bake for 25-30 minutes until topping is golden.

Nutrition Information (per serving):

- Calories: 150
- Protein: 3g
- Carbohydrates: 25g
- Fat: 6g
- Fiber: 5g

- Sugar: 15g

## Coconut Flour Lemon Bars

Ingredients:

- 1 cup coconut flour
- 1/2 cup melted coconut oil
- 1/4 cup honey
- Zest and juice of 2 lemons

Instructions:

1. Preheat the oven to 350°F (175°C).
2. Mix coconut flour, melted coconut oil, honey, lemon zest, and lemon juice.
3. Press into a baking dish and bake for 20-25 minutes.

Nutrition Information (per serving):

- Calories: 130
- Protein: 2g
- Carbohydrates: 15g
- Fat: 8g
- Fiber: 4g
- Sugar: 8g

# Chapter 7: Smoothies

These smoothies not only burst with flavors but also pack a nutritional punch to keep you energized and satisfied. Crafted with a mindful selection of ingredients, each recipe is a delightful blend of taste and health. So, let's embark on a smoothie adventure that's as nourishing as it is delicious.

## Green Detox Smoothie

Ingredients:

- 1 cup spinach
- 1/2 cucumber, peeled
- 1 green apple, cored
- 1/2 lemon, juiced
- 1 cup water
- Ice cubes

Instructions:

1. Combine spinach, cucumber, green apple, and lemon juice in a blender.
2. Add water and blend until smooth.

3. Add ice cubes and blend again for a refreshing touch.

Nutrition Information (per serving):

- Calories: 80
- Protein: 3g
- Carbohydrates: 20g
- Fat: 0.5g
- Fiber: 5g
- Sugar: 10g
- Portion Size: 1 serving

## Berry Blast Smoothie

Ingredients:

- 1/2 cup strawberries, hulled
- 1/2 cup blueberries
- 1/2 cup raspberries
- 1 banana
- 1 cup almond milk
- Ice cubes

Instructions:

1. Combine strawberries, blueberries, raspberries, banana, and almond milk in a blender.
2. Blend until smooth.
3. Add ice cubes and blend again for a refreshing chill.

Nutrition Information (per serving):

- Calories: 120
- Protein: 2g
- Carbohydrates: 30g
- Fat: 1g
- Fiber: 8g
- Sugar: 15g
- Portion Size: 1 serving

## Spinach and Pineapple Smoothie

Ingredients:

- 1 cup fresh pineapple chunks
- 1 cup spinach
- 1/2 banana
- 1/2 cup Greek yogurt
- 1/2 cup water

- Ice cubes

Instructions:

1. Combine pineapple, spinach, banana, Greek yogurt, and water in a blender.
2. Blend until smooth.
3. Add ice cubes and blend again for a tropical twist.

Nutrition Information (per serving):

- Calories: 110
- Protein: 5g
- Carbohydrates: 25g
- Fat: 1g
- Fiber: 4g
- Sugar: 15g
- Portion Size: 1 serving

## Mango Ginger Smoothie

Ingredients:

- 1 cup mango chunks
- 1 tablespoon fresh ginger, grated
- 1/2 cup plain yogurt

- 1/2 cup coconut water
- Ice cubes

Instructions:

1. Combine mango chunks, grated ginger, plain yogurt, and coconut water in a blender.
2. Blend until smooth.
3. Add ice cubes and blend again for a tropical zing.

Nutrition Information (per serving):

- Calories: 130
- Protein: 4g
- Carbohydrates: 30g
- Fat: 1.5g
- Fiber: 3g
- Sugar: 20g
- Portion Size: 1 serving

## Avocado Banana Smoothie

Ingredients:

- 1/2 avocado
- 1 banana

- 1 tablespoon honey

- 1 cup almond milk

- Ice cubes

Instructions:

1. Combine avocado, banana, honey, and almond milk in a blender.

2. Blend until smooth.

3. Add ice cubes and blend again for a creamy delight.

Nutrition Information (per serving):

- Calories: 150

- Protein: 3g

- Carbohydrates: 20g

- Fat: 8g

- Fiber: 6g

- Sugar: 12g

- Portion Size: 1 serving

## Kale and Blueberry Smoothie

Ingredients:

- 1 cup kale, stems removed

- 1/2 cup blueberries

- 1/2 cup plain Greek yogurt

- 1 tablespoon chia seeds

- 1 cup water

- Ice cubes

Instructions:

1. Combine kale, blueberries, Greek yogurt, chia seeds, and water in a blender.

2. Blend until smooth.

3. Add ice cubes and blend again for a nutrient-packed drink.

Nutrition Information (per serving):

- Calories: 100

- Protein: 6g

- Carbohydrates: 18g

- Fat: 2g

- Fiber: 5g

- Sugar: 7g

- Portion Size: 1 serving

# Chocolate Protein Smoothie

Ingredients:

- 1 scoop chocolate protein powder
- 1 tablespoon almond butter
- 1/2 banana
- 1 cup unsweetened almond milk
- Ice cubes

Instructions:

1. Combine chocolate protein powder, almond butter, banana, and almond milk in a blender.
2. Blend until smooth.
3. Add ice cubes and blend again for a protein-packed treat.

Nutrition Information (per serving):

- Calories: 200
- Protein: 20g
- Carbohydrates: 15g
- Fat: 8g
- Fiber: 4g
- Sugar: 6g

- Portion Size: 1 serving

## Peach Almond Smoothie

Ingredients:

- 1 cup sliced peaches
- 1/4 cup almonds
- 1/2 cup vanilla Greek yogurt
- 1/2 cup coconut water
- Ice cubes

Instructions:

1. Combine sliced peaches, almonds, Greek yogurt, and coconut water in a blender.
2. Blend until smooth.
3. Add ice cubes and blend again for a nutty and fruity blend.

Nutrition Information (per serving):

- Calories: 180
- Protein: 7g
- Carbohydrates: 22g
- Fat: 8g

- Fiber: 4g

- Sugar: 16g

- Portion Size: 1 serving

## Citrus Burst Smoothie

Ingredients:

- 1 orange, peeled and segmented

- 1/2 grapefruit, peeled and segmented

- 1/2 cup pineapple chunks

- 1/2 cup plain yogurt

- Ice cubes

Instructions:

1. Combine orange segments, grapefruit segments, pineapple chunks, and plain yogurt in a blender.

2. Blend until smooth.

3. Add ice cubes and blend again for a refreshing burst of citrus.

Nutrition Information (per serving):

- Calories: 110

- Protein: 4g

- Carbohydrates: 25g

- Fat: 1g

- Fiber: 5g

- Sugar: 18g

- Portion Size: 1 serving

## Cucumber Mint Smoothie

Ingredients:

- 1/2 cucumber, peeled

- 1 cup fresh mint leaves

- 1/2 lime, juiced

- 1 cup coconut water

- Ice cubes

Instructions:

1. Combine peeled cucumber, fresh mint leaves, lime juice, and coconut water in a blender.

2. Blend until smooth.

3. Add ice cubes and blend again for a cool and revitalizing experience.

Nutrition Information (per serving):

- Calories: 70

- Protein: 2g

- Carbohydrates: 15g

- Fat: 0.5g

- Fiber: 3g

- Sugar: 8g

- Portion Size: 1 serving

## Tropical Turmeric Smoothie

Ingredients:

- 1/2 cup pineapple chunks

- 1/2 cup mango chunks

- 1/2 teaspoon turmeric powder

- 1 tablespoon flaxseeds

- 1 cup almond milk

- Ice cubes

Instructions:

1. Combine pineapple chunks, mango chunks, turmeric powder, flaxseeds, and almond milk in a blender.

2. Blend until smooth.

3.  Add ice cubes and blend again for a tropical escape.

Nutrition Information (per serving):

- Calories: 120

- Protein: 3g

- Carbohydrates: 20g

- Fat: 5g

- Fiber: 4g

- Sugar: 12g

- Portion Size: 1 serving

## Raspberry Coconut Smoothie

Ingredients:

- 1/2 cup raspberries

- 1/2 cup coconut milk

- 1/2 banana

- 1 tablespoon chia seeds

- Ice cubes

Instructions:

1.  Combine raspberries, coconut milk, banana, and chia seeds in a blender.

2. Blend until smooth.

3. Add ice cubes and blend again for a berry-infused delight.

Nutrition Information (per serving):

- Calories: 130

- Protein: 3g

- Carbohydrates: 18g

- Fat: 7g

- Fiber: 6g

- Sugar: 8g

- Portion Size: 1 serving

## Coffee and Almond Butter Smoothie

Ingredients:

- 1 cup brewed coffee, cooled

- 1 tablespoon almond butter

- 1/2 banana

- 1 tablespoon cocoa powder

- 1 cup unsweetened almond milk

- Ice cubes

Instructions:

1. Combine brewed coffee, almond butter, banana, cocoa powder, and almond milk in a blender.
2. Blend until smooth.
3. Add ice cubes and blend again for a caffeinated and nutty treat.

Nutrition Information (per serving):

- Calories: 90
- Protein: 3g
- Carbohydrates: 15g
- Fat: 4g
- Fiber: 5g
- Sugar: 5g
- Portion Size: 1 serving

## Carrot Cake Smoothie

Ingredients:

- 1/2 cup shredded carrots
- 1/2 banana
- 1/4 cup rolled oats
- 1/2 teaspoon cinnamon

- 1 cup vanilla Greek yogurt
- Ice cubes

Instructions:

1. Combine shredded carrots, banana, rolled oats, cinnamon, and vanilla Greek yogurt in a blender.
2. Blend until smooth.
3. Add ice cubes and blend again for a guilt-free carrot cake indulgence.

Nutrition Information (per serving):

- Calories: 160
- Protein: 10g
- Carbohydrates: 25g
- Fat: 2g
- Fiber: 4g
- Sugar: 12g
- Portion Size: 1 serving

# Mixed Berry Protein Smoothie

Ingredients:

- 1/2 cup mixed berries (strawberries, blueberries, raspberries)
- 1 scoop vanilla protein powder
- 1/2 cup plain Greek yogurt
- 1 tablespoon honey
- 1 cup water
- Ice cubes

Instructions:

1. Combine mixed berries, vanilla protein powder, Greek yogurt, honey, and water in a blender.
2. Blend until smooth.
3. Add ice cubes and blend again for a protein-packed berry sensation.

Nutrition Information (per serving):

- Calories: 140
- Protein: 15g
- Carbohydrates: 20g
- Fat: 2g

- Fiber: 5g
- Sugar: 12g
- Portion Size: 1 serving

# CONCLUSION

As we reach the final chapter of this "Type 2 Diabetes Cookbook for Beginners," it's essential to reflect on the journey we've embarked upon together. This cookbook is not just a compilation of recipes; it's a roadmap towards a healthier, more vibrant life for those managing type 2 diabetes.

In our exploration, we've delved into the intricacies of crafting balanced meals that not only cater to the nutritional needs of diabetes management but also delight the taste buds. The 30-day meal plan serves as a practical guide, offering a structured approach to cultivating sustainable dietary habits.

From the energizing breakfasts that kickstart your day to the satisfying dinners that bring it to a close, each recipe is a testament to the notion that managing diabetes need not be a compromise but an opportunity for culinary creativity. The carefully curated snacks, appetizers, desserts, and smoothies showcase the diversity and richness of flavors available within the bounds of a diabetes-friendly diet.

Beyond the recipes, this book is a companion on your journey to better health. It's a reminder that small, consistent changes can lead to significant transformations. The importance of mindful eating, portion control, and smart food choices is woven into the fabric of every page.

As you conclude this book, remember that this is not an endpoint but a beginning. A beginning of a lifestyle where delicious and nutritious coexist, where every meal is a celebration of well-being. Embrace the knowledge gained, experiment with the recipes, and tailor them to your preferences.

In the spirit of moving forward, let this book be a source of inspiration, empowerment, and motivation. You hold in your hands not just a cookbook but a tool for fostering a positive relationship with food, a key ally in managing type 2 diabetes effectively.

Here's to your health, to the joy of cooking and eating well, and to a future filled with vitality and balance. May your culinary journey be as fulfilling as the meals you create, and may each bite be a step towards a healthier, happier you.